MW01181023

This publication is designed to provide accurate and authoritative information in
regard to the subject matter covered. It is sold the understanding that the publisher
is not engaged in rendering legal, accounting, or other professional services. If
legal advice or other expert assistance is required, the services of a competent
professional person should be sought.

Cover image designed by Freepik.com

First Printing, 2014

Printed in the United States of America

Day / Date:	Hours Slept:

Breakfast	Calories

Lunch	Calories

Dinner	Calories

Snacks	Calories

Glasses of Water: 1 2 3 4 5 6 7 8 | *Total Calories:*

Supplements:

Exercise/Physical Activity:

Notes (energy level, areas of improvement, etc):

Day / Date: | **Hours Slept:**

Breakfast	Calories

Lunch	Calories

Dinner	Calories

Snacks	Calories

Glasses of Water: 1 2 3 4 5 6 7 8 | *Total Calories:*

Supplements:

Exercise/Physical Activity:

Notes (energy level, areas of improvement, etc):

Day / Date:	Hours Slept:

Breakfast	Calories

Lunch	Calories

Dinner	Calories

Snacks	Calories

Glasses of Water: 1 2 3 4 5 6 7 8   *Total Calories:*

Supplements:

Exercise/Physical Activity:

Notes (energy level, areas of improvement, etc):

Day / Date:		Hours Slept:

Breakfast	Calories

Lunch	Calories

Dinner	Calories

Snacks	Calories

Glasses of Water: 1 2 3 4 5 6 7 8   *Total Calories:*

Supplements:

Exercise/Physical Activity:

Notes (energy level, areas of improvement, etc):

Day / Date:	Hours Slept:

Breakfast	Calories

Lunch	Calories

Dinner	Calories

Snacks	Calories

Glasses of Water: 1 2 3 4 5 6 7 8 | *Total Calories:*

Supplements:

Exercise/Physical Activity:

Notes (energy level, areas of improvement, etc):

Day / Date:	Hours Slept:

Breakfast	Calories

Lunch	Calories

Dinner	Calories

Snacks	Calories

Glasses of Water: 1 2 3 4 5 6 7 8   *Total Calories:*

Supplements:

Exercise/Physical Activity:

Notes (energy level, areas of improvement, etc):

Day / Date:		Hours Slept:

Breakfast	Calories

Lunch	Calories

Dinner	Calories

Snacks	Calories

Glasses of Water: 1 2 3 4 5 6 7 8 | *Total Calories:*

Supplements:

Exercise/Physical Activity:

Notes (energy level, areas of improvement, etc):

Day / Date: **Hours Slept:**

Breakfast	Calories

Lunch	Calories

Dinner	Calories

Snacks	Calories

Glasses of Water: 1 2 3 4 5 6 7 8   *Total Calories:*

Supplements:

Exercise/Physical Activity:

Notes (energy level, areas of improvement, etc):

Day / Date:	Hours Slept:	
Breakfast		**Calories**
Lunch		**Calories**
Dinner		**Calories**
Snacks		**Calories**

Glasses of Water: 1 2 3 4 5 6 7 8   *Total Calories:*

Supplements:

Exercise/Physical Activity:

Notes (energy level, areas of improvement, etc):

Day / Date:	Hours Slept:	
Breakfast		**Calories**
Lunch		**Calories**
Dinner		**Calories**
Snacks		**Calories**

Glasses of Water: 1 2 3 4 5 6 7 8   *Total Calories:*

Supplements:

Exercise/Physical Activity:

Notes (energy level, areas of improvement, etc):

Day / Date:		Hours Slept:

Breakfast	Calories

Lunch	Calories

Dinner	Calories

Snacks	Calories

Glasses of Water: 1 2 3 4 5 6 7 8   *Total Calories:*

Supplements:

Exercise/Physical Activity:

Notes (energy level, areas of improvement, etc):

Day / Date: **Hours Slept:**

Breakfast	Calories

Lunch	Calories

Dinner	Calories

Snacks	Calories

Glasses of Water: 1 2 3 4 5 6 7 8   *Total Calories:*

Supplements:

Exercise/Physical Activity:

Notes (energy level, areas of improvement, etc):

Day / Date:	Hours Slept:

Breakfast	Calories

Lunch	Calories

Dinner	Calories

Snacks	Calories

Glasses of Water: 1 2 3 4 5 6 7 8 | *Total Calories:*

Supplements:

Exercise/Physical Activity:

Notes (energy level, areas of improvement, etc):

13

Day / Date: **Hours Slept:**

Breakfast	Calories

Lunch	Calories

Dinner	Calories

Snacks	Calories

Glasses of Water: 1 2 3 4 5 6 7 8   *Total Calories:*

Supplements:

Exercise/Physical Activity:

Notes (energy level, areas of improvement, etc):

Day / Date:	Hours Slept:	
Breakfast		**Calories**
Lunch		**Calories**
Dinner		**Calories**
Snacks		**Calories**

Glasses of Water: 1 2 3 4 5 6 7 8   *Total Calories:*

Supplements:

Exercise/Physical Activity:

Notes (energy level, areas of improvement, etc):

Day / Date:	Hours Slept:	
Breakfast		**Calories**
Lunch		**Calories**
Dinner		**Calories**
Snacks		**Calories**

Glasses of Water: 1 2 3 4 5 6 7 8   *Total Calories:*

Supplements:

Exercise/Physical Activity:

Notes (energy level, areas of improvement, etc):

Day / Date:	Hours Slept:	
Breakfast		**Calories**
Lunch		**Calories**
Dinner		**Calories**
Snacks		**Calories**

Glasses of Water: 1 2 3 4 5 6 7 8   *Total Calories:*

Supplements:

Exercise/Physical Activity:

Notes (energy level, areas of improvement, etc):

17

Day / Date: | **Hours Slept:**

Breakfast	Calories

Lunch	Calories

Dinner	Calories

Snacks	Calories

Glasses of Water: 1 2 3 4 5 6 7 8   *Total Calories:*

Supplements:

Exercise/Physical Activity:

Notes (energy level, areas of improvement, etc):

18

Day / Date:	Hours Slept:

Breakfast	Calories

Lunch	Calories

Dinner	Calories

Snacks	Calories

Glasses of Water: 1 2 3 4 5 6 7 8   *Total Calories:*

Supplements:

Exercise/Physical Activity:

Notes (energy level, areas of improvement, etc):

19

Day / Date: **Hours Slept:**

Breakfast	Calories

Lunch	Calories

Dinner	Calories

Snacks	Calories

Glasses of Water: 1 2 3 4 5 6 7 8   *Total Calories:*

Supplements:

Exercise/Physical Activity:

Notes (energy level, areas of improvement, etc):

Day / Date: | **Hours Slept:**

Breakfast	Calories

Lunch	Calories

Dinner	Calories

Snacks	Calories

Glasses of Water: 1 2 3 4 5 6 7 8 | *Total Calories:*

Supplements:

Exercise/Physical Activity:

Notes (energy level, areas of improvement, etc):

Day / Date:	Hours Slept:

Breakfast	Calories

Lunch	Calories

Dinner	Calories

Snacks	Calories

Glasses of Water: 1 2 3 4 5 6 7 8   *Total Calories:*

Supplements:

Exercise/Physical Activity:

Notes (energy level, areas of improvement, etc):

Day / Date:	Hours Slept:

Breakfast	Calories

Lunch	Calories

Dinner	Calories

Snacks	Calories

Glasses of Water: 1 2 3 4 5 6 7 8   *Total Calories:*

Supplements:

Exercise/Physical Activity:

Notes (energy level, areas of improvement, etc):

Day / Date:	Hours Slept:

Breakfast	Calories

Lunch	Calories

Dinner	Calories

Snacks	Calories

Glasses of Water: 1 2 3 4 5 6 7 8   *Total Calories:*

Supplements:

Exercise/Physical Activity:

Notes (energy level, areas of improvement, etc):

Day / Date:	Hours Slept:

Breakfast	Calories

Lunch	Calories

Dinner	Calories

Snacks	Calories

Glasses of Water: 1 2 3 4 5 6 7 8   *Total Calories:*

Supplements:

Exercise/Physical Activity:

Notes (energy level, areas of improvement, etc):

Day / Date: **Hours Slept:**

Breakfast	Calories

Lunch	Calories

Dinner	Calories

Snacks	Calories

Glasses of Water: 1 2 3 4 5 6 7 8   *Total Calories:*

Supplements:

Exercise/Physical Activity:

Notes (energy level, areas of improvement, etc):

Day / Date:	Hours Slept:

Breakfast	Calories

Lunch	Calories

Dinner	Calories

Snacks	Calories

Glasses of Water: 1 2 3 4 5 6 7 8   *Total Calories:*

Supplements:

Exercise/Physical Activity:

Notes (energy level, areas of improvement, etc):

Day / Date:	Hours Slept:

Breakfast	Calories

Lunch	Calories

Dinner	Calories

Snacks	Calories

Glasses of Water: 1 2 3 4 5 6 7 8	*Total Calories:*

Supplements:

Exercise/Physical Activity:

Notes (energy level, areas of improvement, etc):

Day / Date:	Hours Slept:	
Breakfast		**Calories**
Lunch		**Calories**
Dinner		**Calories**
Snacks		**Calories**

Glasses of Water: 1 2 3 4 5 6 7 8 | *Total Calories:*

Supplements:

Exercise/Physical Activity:

Notes (energy level, areas of improvement, etc):

Day / Date:	Hours Slept:

Breakfast	Calories

Lunch	Calories

Dinner	Calories

Snacks	Calories

Glasses of Water: 1 2 3 4 5 6 7 8   *Total Calories:*

Supplements:

Exercise/Physical Activity:

Notes (energy level, areas of improvement, etc):

Day / Date:	Hours Slept:

Breakfast	Calories

Lunch	Calories

Dinner	Calories

Snacks	Calories

Glasses of Water: 1 2 3 4 5 6 7 8 | *Total Calories:*

Supplements:

Exercise/Physical Activity:

Notes (energy level, areas of improvement, etc):

31

Day / Date: | **Hours Slept:**

Breakfast	Calories

Lunch	Calories

Dinner	Calories

Snacks	Calories

Glasses of Water: 1 2 3 4 5 6 7 8   *Total Calories:*

Supplements:

Exercise/Physical Activity:

Notes (energy level, areas of improvement, etc):

Day / Date:		Hours Slept:	
Breakfast			**Calories**
Lunch			**Calories**
Dinner			**Calories**
Snacks			**Calories**

Glasses of Water: 1 2 3 4 5 6 7 8 *Total Calories:*

Supplements:

Exercise/Physical Activity:

Notes (energy level, areas of improvement, etc):

Day / Date:		Hours Slept:	
Breakfast			**Calories**
Lunch			**Calories**
Dinner			**Calories**
Snacks			**Calories**

Glasses of Water: 1 2 3 4 5 6 7 8   *Total Calories:*

Supplements:

Exercise/Physical Activity:

Notes (energy level, areas of improvement, etc):

Day / Date:	Hours Slept:	
Breakfast		**Calories**
Lunch		**Calories**
Dinner		**Calories**
Snacks		**Calories**

Glasses of Water: 1 2 3 4 5 6 7 8   *Total Calories:*

Supplements:

Exercise/Physical Activity:

Notes (energy level, areas of improvement, etc):

Day / Date:	Hours Slept:	
Breakfast		**Calories**
Lunch		**Calories**
Dinner		**Calories**
Snacks		**Calories**

Glasses of Water: 1 2 3 4 5 6 7 8   *Total Calories:*

Supplements:

Exercise/Physical Activity:

Notes (energy level, areas of improvement, etc):

Day / Date:	Hours Slept:

Breakfast	Calories

Lunch	Calories

Dinner	Calories

Snacks	Calories

Glasses of Water: 1 2 3 4 5 6 7 8 | *Total Calories:*

Supplements:

Exercise/Physical Activity:

Notes (energy level, areas of improvement, etc):

37

Day / Date: **Hours Slept:**

Breakfast	Calories

Lunch	Calories

Dinner	Calories

Snacks	Calories

Glasses of Water: 1 2 3 4 5 6 7 8   *Total Calories:*

Supplements:

Exercise/Physical Activity:

Notes (energy level, areas of improvement, etc):

Day / Date:		Hours Slept:
Breakfast		**Calories**
Lunch		**Calories**
Dinner		**Calories**
Snacks		**Calories**

Glasses of Water: 1 2 3 4 5 6 7 8   *Total Calories:*

Supplements:

Exercise/Physical Activity:

Notes (energy level, areas of improvement, etc):

Day / Date:		Hours Slept:
Breakfast		**Calories**
Lunch		**Calories**
Dinner		**Calories**
Snacks		**Calories**

Glasses of Water: 1 2 3 4 5 6 7 8   *Total Calories:*

Supplements:

Exercise/Physical Activity:

Notes (energy level, areas of improvement, etc):

Day / Date:		Hours Slept:
Breakfast		**Calories**
Lunch		**Calories**
Dinner		**Calories**
Snacks		**Calories**

Glasses of Water: 1 2 3 4 5 6 7 8   *Total Calories:*

Supplements:

Exercise/Physical Activity:

Notes (energy level, areas of improvement, etc):

41

Day / Date: | **Hours Slept:**

Breakfast	Calories

Lunch	Calories

Dinner	Calories

Snacks	Calories

Glasses of Water: 1 2 3 4 5 6 7 8   *Total Calories:*

Supplements:

Exercise/Physical Activity:

Notes (energy level, areas of improvement, etc):

Day / Date:	Hours Slept:

Breakfast	Calories

Lunch	Calories

Dinner	Calories

Snacks	Calories

Glasses of Water: 1 2 3 4 5 6 7 8	*Total Calories:*

Supplements:

Exercise/Physical Activity:

Notes (energy level, areas of improvement, etc):

Day / Date: **Hours Slept:**

Breakfast	Calories

Lunch	Calories

Dinner	Calories

Snacks	Calories

Glasses of Water: 1 2 3 4 5 6 7 8   *Total Calories:*

Supplements:

Exercise/Physical Activity:

Notes (energy level, areas of improvement, etc):

Day / Date:	Hours Slept:	
Breakfast		**Calories**
Lunch		**Calories**
Dinner		**Calories**
Snacks		**Calories**

Glasses of Water: 1 2 3 4 5 6 7 8   *Total Calories:*

Supplements:

Exercise/Physical Activity:

Notes (energy level, areas of improvement, etc):

Day / Date:	Hours Slept:

Breakfast	Calories

Lunch	Calories

Dinner	Calories

Snacks	Calories

Glasses of Water: 1 2 3 4 5 6 7 8 *Total Calories:*

Supplements:

Exercise/Physical Activity:

Notes (energy level, areas of improvement, etc):

Day / Date:	Hours Slept:

Breakfast	Calories

Lunch	Calories

Dinner	Calories

Snacks	Calories

Glasses of Water: 1 2 3 4 5 6 7 8   *Total Calories:*

Supplements:

Exercise/Physical Activity:

Notes (energy level, areas of improvement, etc):

Day / Date: | **Hours Slept:**

Breakfast	Calories

Lunch	Calories

Dinner	Calories

Snacks	Calories

Glasses of Water: 1 2 3 4 5 6 7 8 | *Total Calories:*

Supplements:

Exercise/Physical Activity:

Notes (energy level, areas of improvement, etc):

Day / Date:	Hours Slept:

Breakfast	Calories

Lunch	Calories

Dinner	Calories

Snacks	Calories

Glasses of Water: 1 2 3 4 5 6 7 8 | *Total Calories:*

Supplements:

Exercise/Physical Activity:

Notes (energy level, areas of improvement, etc):

49

Day / Date: **Hours Slept:**

Breakfast	Calories

Lunch	Calories

Dinner	Calories

Snacks	Calories

Glasses of Water: 1 2 3 4 5 6 7 8   *Total Calories:*

Supplements:

Exercise/Physical Activity:

Notes (energy level, areas of improvement, etc):

Day / Date:		Hours Slept:	
Breakfast			**Calories**
Lunch			**Calories**
Dinner			**Calories**
Snacks			**Calories**

Glasses of Water: 1 2 3 4 5 6 7 8   *Total Calories:*

Supplements:

Exercise/Physical Activity:

Notes (energy level, areas of improvement, etc):

Day / Date:	Hours Slept:

Breakfast	Calories

Lunch	Calories

Dinner	Calories

Snacks	Calories

Glasses of Water: 1 2 3 4 5 6 7 8 | *Total Calories:*

Supplements:

Exercise/Physical Activity:

Notes (energy level, areas of improvement, etc):

Day / Date: **Hours Slept:**

Breakfast	Calories

Lunch	Calories

Dinner	Calories

Snacks	Calories

Glasses of Water: 1 2 3 4 5 6 7 8   *Total Calories:*

Supplements:

Exercise/Physical Activity:

Notes (energy level, areas of improvement, etc):

Day / Date:	Hours Slept:

Breakfast	Calories

Lunch	Calories

Dinner	Calories

Snacks	Calories

Glasses of Water: 1 2 3 4 5 6 7 8   *Total Calories:*

Supplements:

Exercise/Physical Activity:

Notes (energy level, areas of improvement, etc):

Day / Date:	Hours Slept:

Breakfast	Calories

Lunch	Calories

Dinner	Calories

Snacks	Calories

Glasses of Water: 1 2 3 4 5 6 7 8   *Total Calories:*

Supplements:

Exercise/Physical Activity:

Notes (energy level, areas of improvement, etc):

Day / Date: Hours Slept:

Breakfast	Calories

Lunch	Calories

Dinner	Calories

Snacks	Calories

Glasses of Water: 1 2 3 4 5 6 7 8   *Total Calories:*

Supplements:

Exercise/Physical Activity:

Notes (energy level, areas of improvement, etc):

Day / Date:	Hours Slept:	
Breakfast		**Calories**
Lunch		**Calories**
Dinner		**Calories**
Snacks		**Calories**

Glasses of Water: 1 2 3 4 5 6 7 8   *Total Calories:*

Supplements:

Exercise/Physical Activity:

Notes (energy level, areas of improvement, etc):

Day / Date:	Hours Slept:

Breakfast	Calories

Lunch	Calories

Dinner	Calories

Snacks	Calories

Glasses of Water: 1 2 3 4 5 6 7 8 | *Total Calories:*

Supplements:

Exercise/Physical Activity:

Notes (energy level, areas of improvement, etc):

Day / Date: | **Hours Slept:**

Breakfast	Calories

Lunch	Calories

Dinner	Calories

Snacks	Calories

Glasses of Water: 1 2 3 4 5 6 7 8 | *Total Calories:*

Supplements:

Exercise/Physical Activity:

Notes (energy level, areas of improvement, etc):

Day / Date: **Hours Slept:**

Breakfast	Calories

Lunch	Calories

Dinner	Calories

Snacks	Calories

Glasses of Water: 1 2 3 4 5 6 7 8   *Total Calories:*

Supplements:

Exercise/Physical Activity:

Notes (energy level, areas of improvement, etc):

Day / Date:		Hours Slept:

Breakfast	Calories

Lunch	Calories

Dinner	Calories

Snacks	Calories

Glasses of Water: 1 2 3 4 5 6 7 8   *Total Calories:*

Supplements:

Exercise/Physical Activity:

Notes (energy level, areas of improvement, etc):

Day / Date: | **Hours Slept:**

Breakfast	Calories

Lunch	Calories

Dinner	Calories

Snacks	Calories

Glasses of Water: 1 2 3 4 5 6 7 8   *Total Calories:*

Supplements:

Exercise/Physical Activity:

Notes (energy level, areas of improvement, etc):

Day / Date:	Hours Slept:

Breakfast	Calories

Lunch	Calories

Dinner	Calories

Snacks	Calories

Glasses of Water: 1 2 3 4 5 6 7 8   *Total Calories:*

Supplements:

Exercise/Physical Activity:

Notes (energy level, areas of improvement, etc):

63

Day / Date:	Hours Slept:

Breakfast	Calories

Lunch	Calories

Dinner	Calories

Snacks	Calories

Glasses of Water: 1 2 3 4 5 6 7 8	*Total Calories:*

Supplements:

Exercise/Physical Activity:

Notes (energy level, areas of improvement, etc):

64

Day / Date:		Hours Slept:
Breakfast		**Calories**
Lunch		**Calories**
Dinner		**Calories**
Snacks		**Calories**

Glasses of Water: 1 2 3 4 5 6 7 8 | *Total Calories:*

Supplements:

Exercise/Physical Activity:

Notes (energy level, areas of improvement, etc):

65

Day / Date: | **Hours Slept:**

Breakfast	Calories

Lunch	Calories

Dinner	Calories

Snacks	Calories

Glasses of Water: 1 2 3 4 5 6 7 8   *Total Calories:*

Supplements:

Exercise/Physical Activity:

Notes (energy level, areas of improvement, etc):

Day / Date:	Hours Slept:

Breakfast	Calories

Lunch	Calories

Dinner	Calories

Snacks	Calories

Glasses of Water: 1 2 3 4 5 6 7 8   *Total Calories:*

Supplements:

Exercise/Physical Activity:

Notes (energy level, areas of improvement, etc):

Day / Date: **Hours Slept:**

Breakfast	Calories

Lunch	Calories

Dinner	Calories

Snacks	Calories

Glasses of Water: 1 2 3 4 5 6 7 8   *Total Calories:*

Supplements:

Exercise/Physical Activity:

Notes (energy level, areas of improvement, etc):

68

Day / Date:	Hours Slept:	
Breakfast		**Calories**
Lunch		**Calories**
Dinner		**Calories**
Snacks		**Calories**

Glasses of Water: 1 2 3 4 5 6 7 8   *Total Calories:*

Supplements:

Exercise/Physical Activity:

Notes (energy level, areas of improvement, etc):

Day / Date:		Hours Slept:

Breakfast	Calories

Lunch	Calories

Dinner	Calories

Snacks	Calories

Glasses of Water: 1 2 3 4 5 6 7 8   *Total Calories:*

Supplements:

Exercise/Physical Activity:

Notes (energy level, areas of improvement, etc):

Day / Date:	Hours Slept:

Breakfast	Calories

Lunch	Calories

Dinner	Calories

Snacks	Calories

Glasses of Water: 1 2 3 4 5 6 7 8   *Total Calories:*

Supplements:

Exercise/Physical Activity:

Notes (energy level, areas of improvement, etc):

Day / Date:	Hours Slept:

Breakfast	Calories

Lunch	Calories

Dinner	Calories

Snacks	Calories

Glasses of Water: 1 2 3 4 5 6 7 8   *Total Calories:*

Supplements:

Exercise/Physical Activity:

Notes (energy level, areas of improvement, etc):

Day / Date:		Hours Slept:

Breakfast	Calories

Lunch	Calories

Dinner	Calories

Snacks	Calories

Glasses of Water: 1 2 3 4 5 6 7 8   *Total Calories:*

Supplements:

Exercise/Physical Activity:

Notes (energy level, areas of improvement, etc):

Day / Date: **Hours Slept:**

Breakfast	Calories

Lunch	Calories

Dinner	Calories

Snacks	Calories

Glasses of Water: 1 2 3 4 5 6 7 8   *Total Calories:*

Supplements:

Exercise/Physical Activity:

Notes (energy level, areas of improvement, etc):

Day / Date:		Hours Slept:

Breakfast	Calories

Lunch	Calories

Dinner	Calories

Snacks	Calories

Glasses of Water: 1 2 3 4 5 6 7 8 | *Total Calories:*

Supplements:

Exercise/Physical Activity:

Notes (energy level, areas of improvement, etc):

75

Day / Date:	Hours Slept:	
Breakfast		**Calories**
Lunch		**Calories**
Dinner		**Calories**
Snacks		**Calories**

Glasses of Water: 1 2 3 4 5 6 7 8   *Total Calories:*

Supplements:

Exercise/Physical Activity:

Notes (energy level, areas of improvement, etc):

Day / Date:	Hours Slept:

Breakfast	Calories

Lunch	Calories

Dinner	Calories

Snacks	Calories

Glasses of Water: 1 2 3 4 5 6 7 8   *Total Calories:*

Supplements:

Exercise/Physical Activity:

Notes (energy level, areas of improvement, etc):

Day / Date:	Hours Slept:

Breakfast	Calories

Lunch	Calories

Dinner	Calories

Snacks	Calories

Glasses of Water: 1 2 3 4 5 6 7 8   *Total Calories:*

Supplements:

Exercise/Physical Activity:

Notes (energy level, areas of improvement, etc):

Day / Date:	Hours Slept:

Breakfast	Calories

Lunch	Calories

Dinner	Calories

Snacks	Calories

Glasses of Water: 1 2 3 4 5 6 7 8   *Total Calories:*

Supplements:

Exercise/Physical Activity:

Notes (energy level, areas of improvement, etc):

79

Day / Date: | **Hours Slept:**

Breakfast	Calories

Lunch	Calories

Dinner	Calories

Snacks	Calories

Glasses of Water: 1 2 3 4 5 6 7 8   *Total Calories:*

Supplements:

Exercise/Physical Activity:

Notes (energy level, areas of improvement, etc):

Day / Date:	Hours Slept:	
Breakfast		**Calories**
Lunch		**Calories**
Dinner		**Calories**
Snacks		**Calories**

Glasses of Water: 1 2 3 4 5 6 7 8   *Total Calories:*

Supplements:

Exercise/Physical Activity:

Notes (energy level, areas of improvement, etc):

Day / Date:		Hours Slept:

Breakfast	Calories

Lunch	Calories

Dinner	Calories

Snacks	Calories

Glasses of Water: 1 2 3 4 5 6 7 8 | *Total Calories:*

Supplements:

Exercise/Physical Activity:

Notes (energy level, areas of improvement, etc):

Day / Date:	Hours Slept:	
Breakfast		**Calories**
Lunch		**Calories**
Dinner		**Calories**
Snacks		**Calories**

Glasses of Water: 1 2 3 4 5 6 7 8   *Total Calories:*

Supplements:

Exercise/Physical Activity:

Notes (energy level, areas of improvement, etc):

Day / Date:	Hours Slept:

Breakfast	Calories

Lunch	Calories

Dinner	Calories

Snacks	Calories

Glasses of Water: 1 2 3 4 5 6 7 8   *Total Calories:*

Supplements:

Exercise/Physical Activity:

Notes (energy level, areas of improvement, etc):

Day / Date:	Hours Slept:

Breakfast	Calories

Lunch	Calories

Dinner	Calories

Snacks	Calories

Glasses of Water: 1 2 3 4 5 6 7 8   *Total Calories:*

Supplements:

Exercise/Physical Activity:

Notes (energy level, areas of improvement, etc):

Day / Date: **Hours Slept:**

Breakfast	Calories

Lunch	Calories

Dinner	Calories

Snacks	Calories

Glasses of Water: 1 2 3 4 5 6 7 8   *Total Calories:*

Supplements:

Exercise/Physical Activity:

Notes (energy level, areas of improvement, etc):

Day / Date:	Hours Slept:	
Breakfast		**Calories**
Lunch		**Calories**
Dinner		**Calories**
Snacks		**Calories**

Glasses of Water: 1 2 3 4 5 6 7 8 *Total Calories:*

Supplements:

Exercise/Physical Activity:

Notes (energy level, areas of improvement, etc):

| Day / Date: | Hours Slept: |

Breakfast	Calories

Lunch	Calories

Dinner	Calories

Snacks	Calories

Glasses of Water: 1 2 3 4 5 6 7 8 **Total Calories:**

Supplements:

Exercise/Physical Activity:

Notes (energy level, areas of improvement, etc):

Day / Date:	Hours Slept:

Breakfast	Calories

Lunch	Calories

Dinner	Calories

Snacks	Calories

Glasses of Water: 1 2 3 4 5 6 7 8   *Total Calories:*

Supplements:

Exercise/Physical Activity:

Notes (energy level, areas of improvement, etc):

Day / Date:	Hours Slept:

Breakfast	Calories

Lunch	Calories

Dinner	Calories

Snacks	Calories

Glasses of Water: 1 2 3 4 5 6 7 8   *Total Calories:*

Supplements:

Exercise/Physical Activity:

Notes (energy level, areas of improvement, etc):

Day / Date:	Hours Slept:

Breakfast	Calories

Lunch	Calories

Dinner	Calories

Snacks	Calories

Glasses of Water: 1 2 3 4 5 6 7 8 | *Total Calories:*

Supplements:

Exercise/Physical Activity:

Notes (energy level, areas of improvement, etc):

Day / Date: **Hours Slept:**

Breakfast	Calories

Lunch	Calories

Dinner	Calories

Snacks	Calories

Glasses of Water: 1 2 3 4 5 6 7 8   *Total Calories:*

Supplements:

Exercise/Physical Activity:

Notes (energy level, areas of improvement, etc):

Day / Date:	Hours Slept:	
Breakfast		**Calories**
Lunch		**Calories**
Dinner		**Calories**
Snacks		**Calories**

Glasses of Water: 1 2 3 4 5 6 7 8   *Total Calories:*

Supplements:

Exercise/Physical Activity:

Notes (energy level, areas of improvement, etc):

Day / Date:	Hours Slept:

Breakfast	Calories

Lunch	Calories

Dinner	Calories

Snacks	Calories

Glasses of Water: 1 2 3 4 5 6 7 8	*Total Calories:*

Supplements:

Exercise/Physical Activity:

Notes (energy level, areas of improvement, etc):

Day / Date: **Hours Slept:**

Breakfast	Calories

Lunch	Calories

Dinner	Calories

Snacks	Calories

Glasses of Water: 1 2 3 4 5 6 7 8   ***Total Calories:***

Supplements:

Exercise/Physical Activity:

Notes (energy level, areas of improvement, etc):

Day / Date:	Hours Slept:

Breakfast	Calories

Lunch	Calories

Dinner	Calories

Snacks	Calories

Glasses of Water: 1 2 3 4 5 6 7 8   *Total Calories:*

Supplements:

Exercise/Physical Activity:

Notes (energy level, areas of improvement, etc):

Day / Date:		Hours Slept:	
Breakfast			**Calories**
Lunch			**Calories**
Dinner			**Calories**
Snacks			**Calories**

Glasses of Water: 1 2 3 4 5 6 7 8   *Total Calories:*

Supplements:

Exercise/Physical Activity:

Notes (energy level, areas of improvement, etc):

Day / Date: **Hours Slept:**

Breakfast   **Calories**

Lunch   **Calories**

Dinner   **Calories**

Snacks   **Calories**

Glasses of Water: 1 2 3 4 5 6 7 8   *Total Calories:*

Supplements:

Exercise/Physical Activity:

Notes (energy level, areas of improvement, etc):

Day / Date:	Hours Slept:	
Breakfast		**Calories**
Lunch		**Calories**
Dinner		**Calories**
Snacks		**Calories**

Glasses of Water: 1 2 3 4 5 6 7 8   *Total Calories:*

Supplements:

Exercise/Physical Activity:

Notes (energy level, areas of improvement, etc):

Day / Date:		Hours Slept:
Breakfast		**Calories**
Lunch		**Calories**
Dinner		**Calories**
Snacks		**Calories**

Glasses of Water: 1 2 3 4 5 6 7 8   *Total Calories:*

Supplements:

Exercise/Physical Activity:

Notes (energy level, areas of improvement, etc):

Day / Date:		Hours Slept:	
Breakfast			**Calories**
Lunch			**Calories**
Dinner			**Calories**
Snacks			**Calories**

Glasses of Water: 1 2 3 4 5 6 7 8   *Total Calories:*

Supplements:

Exercise/Physical Activity:

Notes (energy level, areas of improvement, etc):

More From Recordkeeper Press

Recordkeeper Press would like to thank you for purchasing this product – we hope you love it and use it for years to come!

The Recordkeeper catalog is continually expanding, and contains a wide range of useful and fun products, such as blank recipe books, password journals, and creative notebooks. To browse our other products, you can find our complete online catalog by searching for Recordkeeper Press on Amazon.com.

Thanks again for using our product, and happy record keeping!

CPSIA information can be obtained at www.ICGtesting.com
Printed in the USA
LVOW06s0354221215

467469LV00027B/692/P